Rebuild Your Health with a Mediterranean Diet

Heart Healthy Eating Tips

By Tammy Moore

Legal & Disclaimer

The information contained in this book is not designed to replace or take the place of any form of medicine or professional medical advice. The information in this book has been provided for educational and entertainment purposes only.

The information contained in this book has been compiled from sources deemed reliable, and it is accurate to the best of the Author's knowledge; however, the Author cannot guarantee its accuracy and validity and cannot be held liable for any errors or omissions. Changes are periodically made to this book. You must consult your doctor or get professional medical advice before using any of the suggested remedies, techniques, or information in this book.

Upon using the information contained in this book, you agree to hold harmless the Author from and against any damages, costs, and expenses, including any legal fees potentially resulting from the application of any of the information provided by this guide. This disclaimer applies to any damages or injury caused by the use and application, whether directly or indirectly, of any advice or information presented, whether for breach of contract, tort, negligence, personal injury, criminal intent, or under any other cause of action.

You agree to accept all risks of using the information presented inside this book. You need to consult a professional medical practitioner in order to ensure you are both able and healthy enough to participate in this program.

Table of Contents

INTRODUCTION...1

CHAPTER 1 – AN OVERVIEW OF THE
MEDITERRANEAN DIET......................................3

The worldwide recognition of the Mediterranean diet....5

CHAPTER 2 – THE WAY OF THE
MEDITERRANEAN LIFE......................................8

Foods that are recommended in the Mediterranean Diet 10

CHAPTER 3 – STARTING THE CHANGE TO THE
MEDITERRANEAN WAY OF LIVING.................14

CHAPTER 4 – RECIPES TO HELP YOU LOSE
WEIGHT 17

CHAPTER 5 – RECIPES TO KEEP YOU HEALTHY.32

CONCLUSION...44

Check Out Other Books 45

Introduction

There have been enough fads, methods, and ways of eating introduced in the market for quite some time now. Many claimed that this is the best way to lose weight, live a healthy lifestyle or have a longer life. Not all remained for long, others proved to be effective while others were soon forgotten.

Choosing to eat healthy is a lifestyle and most people desire to lose weight, look good, and of course live a longer life. One of the highly acclaimed methods for eating healthy is the Mediterranean diet. There have been studies, statistics, and proof that this diet really works. Unlike other diets introduced, this diet is not very restrictive and this is the one you can stick with very easily.

Personally, I will tell you that my family is of Italian decent and many of my relatives have lived well past 85 years old. My father's sister lived past her 104th birthday. Since she was 80, I tried to visit her a few times a year. I was living in the northeast of the US and she was living in the warmer weather in the southeast of the US. I started to ask her what her secret was to living so long. As you will read throughout this book many of the tips for a Mediterranean diet are exactly the same things she would tell me for many years. I wish I pay attention to her advice sooner!

Since you are reading this book, it means that you have made a decision to change your life and learn the benefits of this diet. I assure you that you will learn recipes from this book while still enjoying eating tasty and healthy food. In the pages that follow you will find the reasons why this diet works, steps to easily implement it in your life, and the healthy and delicious recipes to change your lifestyle to a common Mediterranean diet. Discover the wonders this diet will bring you and start living healthy today.

I decided to write this book so I could pass on the advice from my aunt and the lessons I learned after researching a Mediterranean diet. Happy reading and good luck in your journey for a whole new you!

Chapter 1 – An overview of the Mediterranean Diet

The Mediterranean diet is a healthy and modern way of eating inspired by the traditional living habits of the people from Greece, Italy, Spain and Southern France. This diet aims to promote health and long life using a specific mix of dietary foods. Mediterranean cuisine has a wide array of food ingredients to choose from. The main food types are fruits, nuts, vegetables, beans, cereal grains, fish and my favorite - olive oil!!

Despite its name, the diet does not mean that it only follows Mediterranean cuisine alone. This only refers to the origin of the diet and does not necessarily mean that you have to eat Greek, Italian, Spanish, or Southern French cuisine entirely.

This diet has been significantly connected with good health, long life and maintaining a healthy heart. In today's modern lifestyle, excessive use of salt in some fast foods and Western style cuisine has been one of the contributing factors to having high blood pressure. In the Mediterranean diet however, one can replace salt through the use of the healthier alternative of herbs and spices. Aside from lessening the negative effects that salt can bring, herbs have been found to provide exciting flavors in many cuisines.

Research has proven that people following the Mediterranean diet are found to have a lower risk of developing heart disease. This is one of the emphasis for following the Mediterranean diet, and one of my main motivations for following the diet. The basic steps to follow are below:

- Use spices and herbs instead of salt to flavor your food.
- eat a lot of fruits and vegetables daily
- eat some poultry and fish about twice a week
- eat less red meat, just a few times each month
- choose products that are made from plant and vegetable oils, like olive oil
- if you want to drink, drink red wine moderately

It's a great idea to have a balanced meal every day, but you don't need to perfect them in your first try. In everything that you do, practice makes perfect and getting acquainted with these healthy foods and lifestyle will come naturally once you get a hang of it.

The worldwide recognition of the Mediterranean diet

The Mediterranean diet was first publicized by Dr. Ancel Keys, an American Scientist in 1975 while he was in Italy. However, the Mediterranean diet failed to gain popularity until around the 1990s where it began to have a following by health conscious people everywhere.

As compared with other diets, the Mediterranean diet had been seen by others as a great mystery because even if the fat consumption is high, the instances of having hypertension, obesity, cardiovascular diseases, diabetes and cancer are significantly lower in the Mediterranean countries as compare to other Western and European countries. In comparison diets from

5

Western and European neighbor countries can include a large amount of butter, red meat, and animal fats, while eating habits of people from Italy, Spain Greece, and Southern France includes eating a lot more fruits and vegetables on a daily basis.

At present, the Mediterranean diet has become more popular in Non-English speaking countries. These countries have adopted this diet regimen in a higher degree and have seen very good results. Additionally, there have been numerous studies showing that this diet can help prevent strokes, diabetes, heart failure and premature death and a nice side effective is the weight loss. This is the reason why many experts are starting to recommend the Mediterranean diet based on how it has proven itself to be beneficial in living a long and healthy life.

As you will learn in the succeeding chapters you will be provided a more detailed understanding about the benefits of the Mediterranean diet and how you can get started. Next you will be provided various healthy, easy, and delicious recipes that you can begin to try out for yourself.

Enjoy the journey to your ultimate destination of a new healthy life style!

Chapter 2 – The Way of the Mediterranean Life

In order to start a certain diet you have to make sure that you are ready and committed in staying with the diet and changing your eating habits into your regular routine. Do not expect that you will have immediate results or it would make you feel better after just a few days. Like any other life style change, this will take some time, patience and focus until you see the results you expect. Be sure to take the time in reviewing the food that are okay for you and check that you don't have any allergies on the specific food groups that are provided in this diet. I also recommend you consult your doctor or even better a dietician just to ensure you do not have any complications. If you are currently under any medication, your doctor or dietician would be able to provide you any advice prior to starting a new diet.

Let's start by reviewing a few guidelines.

The Basics of the Mediterranean Meal Plan

There is no such thing as just "one right way" in implementing this diet. As mentioned in the previous chapter, the diet is not strictly eating cuisines from Mediterranean countries. In all of the studies analyzed, the diet is high in plant

8

foods but low in animal foods, and eating seafood and fish is recommended at least twice a week.

As with other diet regimens, the Mediterranean way of life should be combined with regular exercise and physical activity. This plan can be prepared and adopted slightly differently to suit the needs or preference of any individual. As I learned from my aunt, sharing meals, having fun with other people, and enjoying life is also the best way to make it a regular part of your weekly and monthly routine.

The basics principles to follow are:

- **Eat more of these:** Fruits, vegetables, nuts, legumes, seeds, potatoes, breads, whole grains, herbs, spices, seafood, fish and EVOO (extra virgin olive oil).
- **Eat these in Moderation:** Poultry products, cheese, eggs and yogurt.
- **Try to Rarely Eat these:** Red meats such as lamb, pork and beef.

Avoid these foods:

- **Added sugar:** Candies, soda, sugar sweetened beverages (or diet beverages with sugar substitutes), ice cream, cakes, and table sugar

- **Refined grains:** Pasta made from refined wheat, white bread, etc.
- **Trans-fats:** Found in most processed foods such as oils often used to cook French fries & margarine sticks
- **Refined Oils:** Vegetable Oil, Canola oil, soybean oil, etc.
- **Processed meat:** Hotdogs, hams, sausages, luncheon meats
- **Other processed foods:** Read Labels – many foods that say they are "low-fat" or "low in sugar" may not be. Make sure to check and read labels carefully before buying them. If in doubt best to avoid them.

Foods that are recommended in the Mediterranean Diet

- Plant foods should be eaten more often
- Use fresh fruit for your dessert
- Eat a higher consumption of nuts, beans, seeds, cereals (preferably wheat, barley, oats, brown rice, or corn)
- Main source of dietary fat should be through Olive oil
- Dairy foods should be yogurt (plain yogurt such as Greek Yogurt is best) and cheeses that are lower in fat (mozzarella is one of the better cheeses)

- Eating fish and poultry products in moderation
- No more than 4 eggs per week
- Red meat should be in small amounts every month
- Drinking red wine in moderation

The Mediterranean diet has low saturated fat. It focuses more on monounsaturated fat and have high amounts of dietary fiber. It also consists of legumes like peas, lentils, alfalfa, beans, and chick peas.

Here are some detailed examples of foods that are recommended:

- **Vegetables:** kale, spinach, tomatoes, broccoli, cauliflower, carrots, cucumbers, and Brussels sprouts.
- **Fruits:** bananas, apples, oranges, strawberries, pears, dates, grapes, figs, peaches, and melons.
- **Seeds and nuts:** walnuts, almonds, hazelnuts, cashews, Macadamia nuts, pumpkin seeds, and sunflower seeds.
- **Legumes:** lentils, beans, peas, chickpeas, and peanuts.
- **Tubers:** sweet potatoes, turnips, potatoes, and yams.
- **Whole grains:** whole oats, brown rice, rye, barley, buckwheat, whole grain breads and pasta

11

- **Seafood and fish:** salmon, sardines, trout, mackerel, tuna, oysters, clams, crabs, and mussels.
- **Poultry:** chicken, turkey, and duck (try to avoid the fat and skin)
- **Eggs:** chicken, duck, & quail eggs.
- **Dairy:** plain yogurt, mozzarella cheese, other low fat cheeses
- **Herbs and spices:** basil, mint, sage, nutmeg, rosemary, garlic, & pepper.
- **Healthy fats:** avocados, avocado oil, olives, and extra virgin olive oil.

The key to having good health is the intake of single, fresh, whole ingredient foods which are free from saturated fats and other chemicals.

Water is one of the most essential elements needed in our body. It's pure and has no harmful ingredients that can significantly improve our well-being. Small amounts of red wine are recommended but optional. Tea and coffee can also be taken as long as it's also in moderation and that you should avoid drinking beverages that have a high sugar content.

Benefits of the Mediterranean Diet

Common benefits from following the Mediterranean Diet:

- Helps prevent the risk of having a stroke. Studies show that people who engage in the Mediterranean diet have a better and healthier life. The food in this diet helped in eliminating the chance of experiencing a stroke.
- Reduces the risk of having diabetes, high cholesterol, and high blood pressure which are all connected with cardio-vascular diseases.
- Increase in life expectancy.
- Good for your brain. Eating foods in the diet improves the function of the brain and lowers the risk in having Alzheimer's disease.
- Helps in losing weight and lessens the risk of being obese due to the healthy foods recommended as part of the diet.
- Helps in protecting your bones due to the calcium enriched food included in the diet such as some vegetables, cheese, and yogurt.
- Can slow the aging process due to the consumption of fresh fruits and vegetables.

Chapter 3 – Starting the change to the Mediterranean Way of Living

At this point maybe you still feel uncertain or doubtful in making the change. To provide some encouragement, I have given some useful tips to guide you through the process:

- **Make sure to eat your breakfast:** This is the most important meal of the day and it's highly recommended that you always eat breakfast. Start your day with fresh fruits, fiber rich foods such as whole grains to jump start your day. This is not only healthy but will keep you energized and full for longer.
- **Eat fish and seafood:** Fish like herring, sardines and tuna are all rich in Omega 3 oils. Clams, mussels, and oysters are very good for your heart and your brain.
- **Eat plenty of greens and vegetables:** Try making a simple plate with a few slices of tomatoes and then drizzle it with EVOO (extra virgin olive oil) topped with mozzarella cheese. How about making your pizza with whole grain flour topped with mushrooms, broccoli, & olives

14

instead of sausages or pepperoni? Salads, soups, and vegetable sticks can also be a perfect way of snacking during the day and getting your daily allowance of vegetables.

- **Eat small amounts of meat:** Though it's really hard to avoid meat, try making the adjustment in a few steps. Avoid red meats and replace them with white meat. Should you sometimes eat those red meat, make sure that you choose lean cuts without all the fat. Then have few servings of white meat each week and only 1-2 servings of red meat per month.
- **Make it a habit to use "good" fat:** EVOO, sunflower seeds, olives, nuts and avocados are great sources of good fat. Use good oils to replace those oils with high polyunsaturated fats like vegetable oil or canola oil.
- **Have a vegetarian meal at least once a week:** Preparing "meatless meals" every once in a while will boost your intake of veggies. This is also a good way to get used to a more vegetarian diet schedule over time.
- **Eat fresh fruits for your dessert**: Instead of sweets such as cake or ice cream, is easy to replace them with fresh fruits like strawberries, bananas, blueberries, apples or grapes. Fruits have natural sugars

15

which is much better than refined sugar you get in cakes and ice cream.

- **Have some dairy products:** You can still enjoy having a dose of dairy products such as plain yogurt or low-fat cheeses.

Chapter 4 – Recipes to Help you Lose Weight

By now you already have an idea on how the Mediterranean diet works and what are the foods you need to include in your everyday diet. Of course, the best way to make this diet work is for you to prepare your own meals. Here are some of the best recipes that will help you lose weight. Put on your cooking hats and aprons, and let's enjoy cooking these mouth-watering Mediterranean recipes!

Sautéed Polenta with Butter Beans

Ingredients

- 4 teaspoons of EVOO (Extra Virgin Olive Oil & divide it)
- 1 16-oz container of prepared plain polenta (those that are in a tube and cut it into ½ inch cubes)
- 1 clove of garlic (minced)
- 1 small onion (cut into half and sliced thinly)
- 1 red bell pepper (diced)
- ½ a teaspoon of smoked paprika
- 1 can of 15-oz butter beans (rinsed)
- 4 cups of baby spinach
- ¾ cup of vegetable broth

- ½ cup of shredded cheese (either Monterey Jack or Manchego)
- 2 teaspoons of sherry vinegar

Directions
1. Over medium heat, add 2 teaspoons of EVOO in a large pan. Add polenta and start cooking around 8-10 minutes, stirring it occasionally until it turns brown. Transfer to a plate and set aside.
2. Reduce heat and add remaining EVOO and sauté garlic. Cook until fragrant then add the bell pepper and onion stirring the mixture occasionally. Add the beans, spinach, and then the vegetable broth. Cook thoroughly until the spinach and beans are done (my aunt will say al dente or slightly crisp, starting to get soft). Remove from the heat and add the cheese and vinegar. Serve it over the polenta and optionally sprinkle with paprika to your taste.

Tips and notes:
Smoked paprika comes in 3 varieties which is hot, sweet or bittersweet. Choose the one that best suits your taste. You can find them in any well-known supermarkets or specialty stores in your area.

Chickpea and Lamb (or Chicken) Soup

Ingredients

For the soup:

- ¾ cup of dried chickpeas (rinsed)
- 3 teaspoons of EVOO (Extra Virgin Olive Oil & divide it)
- 1 large chopped onion
- 2 medium diced carrots
- 3 cloves of minced garlic
- 2 teaspoons of ground cumin
- 1 teaspoon of ground coriander
- ¼ teaspoon of cayenne pepper
- 1 lb. trimmed lamb shank (or chicken thigh or breast)
- 1/8 teaspoon of salt
- ¼ teaspoon of fresh ground pepper
- 4 cups of chicken broth (get the reduced sodium variety)
- 1 14-oz can of diced tomatoes
- 2 pieces of bay leaf
- ½ cup of rinsed bulgur (dried cracked wheat)
- 2 tablespoons of lemon juice

For the Pistachio Mint Pesto:

- 1 & ½ cups of mint leaves (fresh)
- 1/3 cup of shelled pistachios
- 2 cloves of crushed and peeled garlic
- 2 tablespoons of EVOO (extra virgin olive oil)
- 2 tablespoons of lemon juice
- 2 tablespoons of yogurt (low-fat variety)
- 1/8 teaspoon of salt (this is optional)

Directions

1) In preparing the soup, put the chickpeas in a huge bowl. Add water to cover and soak it for about 8-24 hours. You can also choose to cook the chickpeas around 2 minutes in a large saucepan. Then remove from heat and set aside for about an hour, then drain.
2) Heat 2 teaspoons of oil in a large pressure cooker or a 4-quart (large) cooking pot on medium to high heat. Add carrots, onions and cook thoroughly for about 3-5 minutes until soft. Put the cumin, garlic, cayenne and coriander then stir until fragrant. Remove and set aside.
3) Season lamb shank (or chicken) with pepper and salt. Over medium to high heat, add the remaining oil in a medium pan or cast iron skillet then cook the lamb shank (or chicken) turning it over occasionally until seared on both sides. Transfer the shank (or chicken) over to

the pressure cooker or large pot and add the broth, bay leaves, chickpeas and tomatoes. Secure and cover the pressure cooker (or large pot) and cook it over medium to high heat. Cook for about 35 minutes.

4) Place the bulgur in a medium sized bowl. Cover it with boiling water. Let stand for about 15 minutes then drain in sieve making sure to remove excess water.

5) After cooking the shank (or chicken) in the pressure cooker, release the heat on its own. Wait for about 5-20 minutes.

6) For the pesto, use a food processor to finely chop the pistachios, garlic, and mint. Add lemon juice, yogurt, and oil into the feed tube continuously, forming a paste. You may add salt if desired, or if you are using unsalted pistachios.

7) Discard the bay leaves once the pressure has dissipated. Skim the fat from the soup's surface and take the lamb shank with tongs onto a clean, dry cutting board. Before returning the meat into the soup, remember to shred it coarsely once its temperature is cool enough. Heat through after adding the drained bulgur. Pour in the lemon juice and stir. Serve with pesto and enjoy!

Tips and notes:

Bulgur can be made by either drying & coarsely grinding, cracking the wheat berries or parboiling. Cracked wheat is different from bulgur because bulgur can be soaked quickly in hot water while cracked wheat needs to be cooked for about an hour. You can find bulgur in the natural food section or grain section in any well-known large supermarkets.

Tomato Olive Stuffed Portobello Mushroom Caps

Ingredients

- 2/3 cups of plum tomatoes (chopped)
- ½ cup of part skimmed mozzarella cheese (shredded)
- 1 teaspoon of garlic (minced)
- ¼ cup of Kalamata olives (chopped)
- 2 teaspoons of EVOO (extra virgin olive oil, divided)
- ½ teaspoon of fresh rosemary (finely chopped or you can also use 1/8 teaspoon of dried rosemary)
- 1/8 teaspoon of fresh ground pepper
- 4 pieces of Portobello mushroom caps (5 inches wide)
- 2 tablespoons of lemon juice
- 2 teaspoons of soy sauce (reduced-sodium)

Directions

1) In a small sized bowl, combine cheese, olives, tomatoes, garlic, 1 teaspoon of EVOO, pepper, and rosemary.
2) Preheat your grill to medium-high temperature.
3) Cut stems of the mushrooms and using your spoon remove the brown gills under its cap. Throw the gills with the existing mix and the last teaspoon of EVOO, soy sauce and lemon juice in another small bowl. Brush both sides of caps with the mixture and place them on the oiled grill to cook. Grill and cover until cooked for about 5 minutes on each side. Once it is cooked, remove from the grill. Fill the caps with the remaining tomato mix, return it on the grill, cover, and cook completely. Make sure that the cheese is also completely melted for about 3 minutes.
4) Serve hot and enjoy!

Tips and notes:
You can also use scallops for this dish instead of shrimp. When oiling your grill rack, fold a paper towel, add some oil, hold it using tongs and rub the rack with it. Never use any cooking spray over a hot grill as the spray could be flammable.

Toast with Broccoli Rabe, Chicken, & Feta Cheese

Ingredients

- 4 slices of whole wheat bread (thickly sliced)
- 1 clove of garlic (peeled, this is optional)
- ¼ cup of garlic (chopped)
- 4 teaspoons of EVOO (extra virgin olive oil, divided)
- 1 lb. of chicken tenders (cut to crosswise into ½ inch pieces)
- 1 bunch of broccoli rabe (trim the stems and cut into ½ inch pieces)
- 2 cups of cherry tomatoes (halved)
- 1 teaspoon of vinegar (red wine variety)
- 1/8 teaspoon of salt
- Ground pepper (fresh)
- ¾ cup of feta cheese (crumbled)

Directions

1) Toast or grill the bread then rub it lightly with the garlic clove. This is optional. After rubbing with garlic, discard the clove.
2) In a large nonstick pan, add 2 teaspoons of EVOO over medium-high heat. Add the chicken and cook thoroughly for

24

about 4-5 minutes. Transfer the chicken and all its juices on a plate and cover it to keep warm. Set aside.

3) Add remaining EVOO in the pan. Sauté the garlic and cook until translucent and fragrant. Add the broccoli rabe and stir until cooked through. You should be able to see that it's cooked when the broccoli rabe is already bright green and quite wilted. Combine with the tomatoes, salt, pepper, and vinegar. Stir occasionally until tomatoes break down. Return the chicken together with its juices into the pan. Stir in the feta cheese and cook thoroughly.

4) Serve with the garlic toast.

Tips and notes:

You can replace the broccoli rabe with broccolini. This is a sweet and tender vegetable that resembles Chinese kale and broccoli. Broccoli rabe is mildly bitter but pleasantly pungent. It's a part of the cabbage family and is very much used in Mediterranean cuisines.

25

Salad Niçoise with Grilled Halibut

Ingredients

For the vinaigrette:

- 1 clove of garlic (medium sized)
- 5 tablespoons of EVOO
- 6 tablespoons of orange juice (freshly squeezed, add more juice to taste)
- ¼ cup of vinegar (either red wine or white wine variety)
- ½ teaspoon of salt (divided)
- 1 tablespoon of Dijon mustard

For the salad

- 1 & ½ lb. of red potatoes (around 5-6 medium size; cleaned and scrubbed)
- 1 & ¼ lb. of green beans (trimmed)
- 1 piece of large lemon (juiced)
- 2 tablespoons of EVOO (extra virgin olive oil)
- ½ teaspoon of salt (divided)
- 1 lb. of fish (either the Stripped Bass or Pacific Halibut)
- ¼ teaspoon of ground pepper
- 1 piece of large lettuce
- 1 & ½ cups of grape tomatoes

- 3 pieces of eggs (hard-boiled, peeled, cut into wedges)
- ¼ cup of Kalamata olives or black Niçoise (sliced and pitted)
- ¼ cup of fresh parsley (finely chopped)

Directions

1) To prepare the vinaigrette, peel and crush the garlic. In a small bowl, mash garlic using a fork with ¼ teaspoon of salt to make a coarse paste. Whisk 5 tablespoons of oil then add 6 tablespoons of orange juice, mustard, and the vinegar. Continue whisking until combined thoroughly. Taste and add more orange juice to mellow down the flavor to your own taste. Season with salt and set aside.

2) For the salad, bring water to a boil in a large, deep saucepan. Make sure that it would fit in a steamer basket. Add the potatoes and cook until it's tender. Remove and let cool. Once potatoes are cooled, cut and place them in a shallow

bowl. Drizzle it with the prepared 1/3 cup of vinaigrette and set aside.

3) Add the beans inside the steamer basket and cook until it turns bright green and tender. Rinse with cold water and drain well. Put them in a medium bowl then add 2 tablespoons of vinaigrette.

4) Combine the lemon juice, oil, and salt in a re-sealable plastic container. Shake and add the fish to be marinated for about 20 minutes.

5) Preheat the grill to high for about 10 minutes. If you are using a charcoal grill, make sure that the flames subside first because if you cook the fish with flames, this would cause the fish to easily burn.

6) Drain and pat the fish dry. Season it with salt and pepper then oil the grill rack. Place the fish on the grill until both sides are browned and thoroughly cooked. If you are using halibut, grill it for about 4-5 minutes per side while for seabass, it's about 3-4 minutes.

7) On a serving platter, arrange the lettuce leaves and place the fish, green beans, potatoes, and tomatoes on top. With the remaining vinaigrette, drizzle it on top

and garnish with olives, eggs, parsley,
and pepper.
8) Serve and enjoy.

Tips and notes:

In cooking hard-boiled eggs, place the eggs in a medium saucepan and bring water to boil over high heat. Once water is boiling, turn off the heat, cover for about 1-2 minutes. Hot water will continuously cook the eggs until it becomes hard boiled. After a while, remove from hot water and place in cold water to cool. Once cooled, you can handle and peel the eggs.

Mediterranean wrap

Ingredients
- ½ cup of water
- 1/3 cup of couscous (preferably whole wheat)
- 1 cup of fresh parsley (chopped)
- ½ cup of fresh mint (chopped)

- ¼ cup of lemon juice
- 3 tablespoons of EVOO (extra-virgin olive oil)
- 2 teaspoons of garlic (minced)
- ¼ teaspoon of salt (divided)
- ¼ teaspoon of ground pepper (fresh)
- 1 lb. of chicken tenders
- 1 medium tomato (chopped)
- 1 cup cucumber (chopped)
- 4 (10 inch) sun dried tomato (or spinach) wraps (you could also use tortilla)

Directions
1) Add water in a saucepan and bring to a boil. Stir in the couscous and remove from heat. Cover and let it stand for about 5 minutes. Fluff the couscous using a fork. Set aside.
2) In a small bowl, mix mint, parsley, lemon juice, garlic, oil, salt, and pepper.
3) Toss the chicken tenders with a tablespoon of the parsley mixture and salt. Heat a large nonstick pan and cook the chicken tenders over medium to low heat. Transfer to a plate and let cool. Once cooled cut into bite sized pieces and set aside.
4) Add the remaining parsley mixture to the couscous with the cucumber and tomato.
5) Assemble the wraps by spreading about ¾ cups of couscous mixture on it. Put some chicken on each wraps. Roll each wraps

like a burrito and tuck each side in order to hold the filling. Serve immediately and enjoy!

Tips and notes: You can save the leftovers to be wrapped the next day. It's fast, quick, and can be eaten as lunch or dinner. Add some salad greens for a more complete and fuller meal.

Chapter 5 – Recipes to keep you healthy

As mentioned in the previous chapter, one of the benefits of following the Mediterranean diet is having a long and healthy life simply from eating a lot of veggies, minimizing the use of salt in your cooking, and due to the use of the olive oil used in cooking. Here are some more recipes for you to try out and make you feel healthier.

Mediterranean Tuna

Ingredients

- 2 cans of 6-oz tuna (in spring water is best), flaked and drained
- ¼ cup of EVOO (extra virgin olive oil)
- ¼ cup of ripe olives (pitted and chopped)
- ¼ cup of roasted red bell peppers (drained and chopped) (optional)
- 2 green onions (sliced)
- 1 tablespoon of capers (rinsed and drained) (or cashew nuts)
- 6 slices of whole wheat bread

Directions
1) In a medium bowl, combine all of the ingredients except the slices of bread. Mix thoroughly.

2) Arrange over greens, if desired. Serve it with the bread and enjoy!

Tips and notes:
Mediterranean classic ingredients are used in this recipe to create a bold and flavorful combination. You can use this as a spread on any breads or crackers. What's more, no need to spend a lot on tuna because for either fresh or canned tuna – both are packed with Omega 3 fatty acids which is good for your heart.

Skewer Appetizers with Bloody Mary Vinaigrette

Ingredients
- ½ cup of tomato juice
- 2 tablespoons of vodka
- 1/8 teaspoon of Worcestershire sauce
- 2 hearts of celery (finely diced, about 3 tablespoons)
- ¼ teaspoon of seat salt
- ¼ teaspoon of ground black pepper
- Grape tomatoes, Kalamata olives, Bocconcini (mozzarella balls) and artichoke hearts (approx. 32 pieces each)
- 1/8 teaspoon of hot sauce
- ¼ teaspoon of horseradish (prepared)
- 2 tablespoons of EVOO (extra virgin olive oil)

Directions

1) Whisk together vodka, tomato juice, Worcestershire sauce, horseradish, hot sauce, salt, pepper and celery. Mix thoroughly. Set aside and refrigerate.
2) Skewer the tomato, olives, bocconcini, and artichoke hearts. Arrange on a platter and serve with the vinaigrette. Enjoy!

Tips and notes:
This appetizer contains around 150 calories per serving. It's simple, healthy and easy to prepare. You can make the vinaigrette ahead of time and store it in the refrigerator for a few days.

Grilled Seafood with Skordalia Dip

Ingredients
- 1 lb. potatoes (choose either Yukon gold or Russet)
- 8 cloves of garlic (peeled)
- 1 slice of sourdough bread (remove the crust)
- ¼ cup of plain yogurt (low fat Greek variety)
- 3 tablespoons of EVOO (extra virgin olive oil, divided)
- 1 lemon - zest and juice
- ½ teaspoon of salt (divided)
- ¼ teaspoon of dried thyme
- 1 lb. of halibut fillets (separated into 4 pieces)
- 2 red bell peppers (quartered)

- 1 lb. of zucchini (cut diagonally about an inch long pieces)
- ½ red onion (sliced)

Directions

1) Peel the potatoes and cut them to 1 inch pieces. Place them on a large saucepan with cold water and add the garlic. Cover and cook on high heat for approximately 15 minutes or until potatoes are thoroughly cooked.

2) Tear the bread into 3-4 pieces and put them in a large bowl. Scoop around 2-3 tablespoons of water from the saucepan with the cooked potatoes and add them over the bread. Stir using a fork until it becomes smooth. Add the yogurt, lemon juice and zest and 2 tablespoons of oil until it forms into a smooth paste. Set aside.

3) Once potatoes are cooked, drain, and reserve the broth. Transfer the potatoes into the bread mixture and mash until it becomes smooth. Usually a potato riser is the best equipment for this job. Add about 2 tablespoons of the reserved broth slowly until it takes the consistency of mashed potatoes. Add a teaspoon of salt and 2 teaspoons of EVOO. Cover and keep it warm.

4) Preheat a grill pan over medium heat. Drizzle the fish fillets with ½ a teaspoon

of EVOO and season with remaining salt and add thyme. Cook the fish for about 2-3 minutes on each of the side or until fork tender. Transfer into a plate and cover to keep warm.

5) In a large bowl, combine zucchini, bell peppers, and red onion. Drizzle with the remaining ½ a teaspoon of EVOO. Toss lightly to evenly coat the veggies. Cook the veggies on the grill pan for around 10 minutes or until tender.

6) Once done, arrange the cooked ingredients on a plate. Serve with the prepared Skordalia sauce on the side. Enjoy!

Tips and notes:
Skordalia is a Greek dipping sauce that is made with garlic, olive oil, and potatoes. You can use any fish on this recipe, whichever is available or whatever you prefer.

Detox Mediterranean Salad

Ingredients
- 1 8-oz English cucumber
- 2 tablespoons of lemon juice (fresh)
- 2 tablespoons of EVOO (extra virgin olive oil)
- Black pepper for tasting
- 6 cups of watercress (trimmed)

- 1 14-oz can of artichoke hearts (quartered and drained)
- 2 stalks of celery, large (sliced)
- ½ cup of red onion (sliced)
- ½ cup of feta cheese

Directions
1) Cut the cucumber into half then slice it crosswise into ¼ inch thick pieces. Process the ¾ cup of cucumber with the lemon juice in a blender. Add the olive oil and pulse until thoroughly combined. Season with black pepper and transfer the mixture to a large bowl.
2) In a separate bowl, mix in the remaining 1 cup of cucumber, artichoke hearts, celery, watercress, feta cheese, and onion. Drizzle with the dressing mixture and toss evenly.
3) Divide and serve. Enjoy!

Tips and notes:
Cucumbers are considered a super food in the Mediterranean because they are low in calories, and provides a lot of Vitamin K and Vitamin C.

Baked Salmon

Ingredients
- ¼ teaspoon of salt
- ¼ teaspoon of black pepper

- 4 6-oz salmon fillets (about an inch thick and skinless)
- Cooking spray
- 2 cups of cherry tomatoes (slice in half)
- ½ cup of zucchini (finely chopped)
- 2 tablespoons of capers (undrained)
- 1 tablespoon of olive oil
- 1 (2 ¼-oz) can of ripe olives (sliced and drained)

Directions
1) Preheat the oven to 425 degrees.
2) Season the fish with salt and pepper on both sides. Place it on a single layered 11x7 inch baking tray and coat it with cooking spray (or you can use cooking paper).
3) Mix tomatoes, zucchini, capers, and olive oil in a small bowl. Mix thoroughly then add the mixture over the fish. Bake for about 22 minutes.
4) Once done, serve and enjoy!

Tips and notes:
Salmon (one of my Father's, Aunt's, & my favorite fish) is full of mono-saturated fats and a great source of Omega 3 fatty acids which is great for your heart.

Couscous and Veggie Paella

Ingredients
- 2 & ½ tablespoons of olive oil
- 2 cups of onion (chopped)
- 1 cup of red bell pepper (chopped)
- 1 cup of green bell pepper (chopped)
- 1 tablespoon of garlic (chopped)
- 1 & ½ teaspoons of paprika
- 2 cups of vegetable broth (canned)
- 3 plum tomatoes (large size, seeded and coarsely chopped)
- 1 cup of frozen peas
- 1 cup of canned chickpeas (drained)
- ½ cup of carrots (peeled and chopped)
- ¼ teaspoon of cayenne pepper
- ¼ teaspoon of saffron threads (crushed)
- 1 & ½ cups of couscous
- 6 cans of hearts of artichoke (quartered)
- 1 Red bell pepper (sliced into rings)
- 1 piece of lemon (cut into 8 wedges)
- Fresh parsley (chopped)

Directions
1) In a large and heavy pot, heat the oil over medium to high heat. Add the bell peppers and onions. Sauté for about 5 minutes until veggies are cooked well. Add in the paprika and garlic and sauté for another minute. Stir the broth in and add the tomatoes, peas, chickpeas, carrots, saffron threads, and cayenne pepper. Simmer and reduce the heat.

39

Cook for about 5 minutes and season to taste.

2) Mix the couscous with the vegetables. Cook and simmer for a minute. Remove the pot from the heat and let stand for about 5 minutes.

3) Fluff the couscous using a fork. Cover and let it stand for another 5 minutes then fluff it again using the fork. Season with pepper to taste.

4) Transfer to a serving bowl. Arrange with the red bell pepper rings, artichoke hearts, and lemon wedges on top of the vegetable paella. Sprinkle some parsley.

5) Serve and enjoy!

Tips and notes:
Saffron provides a hint of authenticity to the dish as this gets an inspiration from Spain's paella dishes. You can serve green salad with this dish and enjoy a bottle of red wine with your loved one.

White Bean Salad with Grilled Shrimp

Ingredients

- 1 teaspoon of lemon zest
- 1/3 cup of lemon juice
- 3 tablespoons of EVOO (extra virgin olive oil)
- 2 tablespoons of minced oregano (fresh)
- 2 tablespoons of minced sage (fresh)

- 2 tablespoons of minced chives (fresh)
- 1 teaspoon of ground pepper
- ½ teaspoon of sea salt
- 2 (15-oz) canned cannellini beans (rinsed)
- 12 pieces of cherry tomatoes (quartered)
- 1 cup of celery (diced finely)
- 24 pieces of medium sized shrimp (peeled, deveined)

Directions

1) Using a large-sized bowl, combine the oil, oregano, lemon zest, chives, sage, lemon juice, sea salt, and pepper. Mix well and reserve about 2 tablespoons of this mixture in a separate small sized bowl.
2) Add tomatoes, celery, and beans in another large-sized bowl then toss well. Set aside.
3) Meanwhile prepare your grill and pre-heat to medium to high heat. You can also use an electric grill but you don't need to place your shrimp on a skewer.
4) If using a grill, thread shrimps to 6 skewers. Oil grill rack and grill shrimps for around 2 minutes on one side until they turn pink. Turn on the other side and cook for another 2 minutes.
5) Plate the white bean salad and put grilled shrimp on top. Drizzle using the reserved salad dressing mixture. Serve and enjoy!

Tips and notes:

You can also use scallops for this dish instead of shrimp. When oiling your grill rack, fold a paper towel, add some oil, hold it using tongs and rub the rack with it. Never use any cooking spray over a hot grill as the spray could be flammable.

Greek Salad in a Pita

Ingredients

- 3 tablespoons of EVOO (extra virgin olive oil)
- 1 tablespoon of vinegar (use red wine)
- 1 & ¼ cups of tomatoes (you can use cherry or plum; seed and chop)
- 1 cup of cucumber (peeled, diced, and seeded)
- 1 cup of green bell pepper (chopped)
- 2/3 cup of onion (red)
- ½ cup of radish (chopped)
- ½ cup of Italian parsley (fresh and chopped)
- 1 cup of feta cheese (crumbled)
- 4 pieces of 8-inch diameter pita bread (whole wheat; sliced in half)
- Pepper and sea salt for tasting

Directions

1) Using a large-sized bowl, whisk the olive oil and vinegar. Season with pepper and sea salt.
2) Mix in the cucumber, tomatoes, onion, radish, bell pepper and parsley. Add in the feta cheese.
3) Using a slotted spoon, fill in the pita with the salad mixture. Serve sandwiches immediately. Enjoy!

Tips and notes:

You can make the salad two days ahead of time. Just cover it up and chill inside the refrigerator. Once ready to use, just bring it out and you will have instant sandwiches!

Conclusion

As you can tell the Mediterranean diet is a nice alternative to making life healthier. In so many ways, it proves to be a valuable diet plan that every individual can easily learn, and more importantly adopt into their lifestyle. Today's society has changed and is very challenging. With people becoming so busy with work and being stressed all the time, it has become more difficult to watch the food we eat that cares for our body's well-being. Many people fall prey to fast foods, instant foods, and develop bad habits like drinking, smoking, or worse, doing drugs.

To finally come up with this book is an achievement and is my little way of teaching people what I learned from my Aunt and my family of how to live a healthier lifestyle. I would like to thank you for reading this book and I hope that you have been enlightened and begun to learn some recipes that will help you with the steps toward living a healthier and longer life. It is my hope that you will also share this message with others and start prepare these delicious recipes or similar recipes you may learn to create on your own with your family. Teach your whole family how easy it is to eat and reap the benefits of a Mediterranean diet and stay healthier together.

Again my heartfelt gratitude and I hope you will enjoy this book as much as I've enjoyed sharing it with you.

One last favor, if you really liked the book, please leave a review on Amazon.com, and look for my other books on Amazon.

Grazie amici miei!

Check Out Other Books

Take Charge of Your Health

also by **Tammy Moore**